MAYR DIET AFTER 50:

HOW TO LOSE WEIGHT, FEEL YOUNGER AND ENERGIZED, AND PREVENT DISEASES WITH A SIMPLE MEAL PLAN FOR BEGINNERS

Table of Contents

INTRODUCTION 3

CHAPTER 1: BREAKFAST 6

    CLASSIC WESTERN OMELET 6
    TOMATO MOZZARELLA EGG MUFFINS 8
    CRISPY CHAI WAFFLES 9
    THREE CHEESE EGG MUFFINS 12
    ANTI-INFLAMMATORY ENERGY BARS 13
    LEEK & SPINACH FRITTATA 15
    CHERRY CHIA OATS 17
    OVEN-POACHED EGGS 18
    CRANBERRY AND RAISINS GRANOLA 20
    SPICY MARBLE EGGS 22

CHAPTER 2: LUNCH 24

    FARRO SALAD WITH ARUGULA 24
    STIR-FRIED FARROS 26
    CAULIFLOWER BROCCOLI MASH 28
    BROCCOLI AND BLACK BEANS STIR FRY 29
    MUSHROOM "CHICKEN TENDERS" 31
    QUINOA PASTA WITH TOMATO ARTICHOKE SAUCE 33
    ALKALIZING TAHINI NOODLE BOWL 35
    ROASTED VEGETABLES 36
    SWEET AND SOUR ONIONS 39
    SAUTÉED APPLES AND ONIONS 40
    ZUCCHINI NOODLES WITH PORTABELLA MUSHROOMS 42
    GRILLED TEMPEH WITH PINEAPPLE 44
    ALKALINE MEATLOAF 47

CHAPTER 3: DINNER RECIPES 49

    ITALIAN LEEK FRY 49
    BELL PEPPERS & ZUCCHINI STIR FRY 51
    YELLOW SQUASH & BELL PEPPER BAKE 53
    VEGETABLE MEDLEY SAUTÉ 54

CHICKPEA BUTTERNUT SQUASH	56
GRILLED VEGETABLE STACK	58
DATE NIGHT CHIVE BAKE	59
CURRIED ZUCCHINI	61

CHAPTER 4: SALADS 63

BUCKWHEAT SALAD	63
MIXED SPROUTS SALAD	65
THAI QUINOA SALAD	66
SWEET POTATO SALAD	69
WALDORF SALAD	71
ITALIAN ROASTED VEGETABLE SALAD	73
KALE AND CARROT SALAD	75
CAULIFLOWER AND CHERRY TOMATO SALAD	76
WATERMELON SALAD	77
ORANGE CELERY SALAD	78
CAULIFLOWER & TOMATO SALAD	80

CHAPTER 5: DESSERTS AND SNACKS 81

WATERMELON SORBET	81
ALMOND BUTTER BALLS VEGAN	82
COFFEE CREAM	84
ALMOND COOKIES	85
CHOCOLATE MOUSSE	87
STRAWBERRY GRANITA	88
APPLE FRITTERS	90
CHOCOLATE MOUSSE	93

CONCLUSION 95

Introduction

Autoimmune diseases and mental health are treated in the traditional medical community, but they are not *cured*. As we know, treating an illness is a lot more profitable than curing it. There are different ways to alleviate a symptom, but if the root cause is not being addressed, relapse will occur. Having a label placed on you, like bipolar disorder, gives the perception that you have a lifelong condition that cannot be corrected, a condition that can only be treated with pharmaceuticals. Fortunately, this is not the case. In fact, change can occur in a matter of weeks. When referring to the gut, it is estimated that it takes about six weeks for the lining to be completely replaced by new cells. We should not allow ourselves to be categorized under an inescapable label or condition. Instead, we can take responsibility and control the way we take care of ourselves and our microbiota.The following chapters will discuss the basics of the mayr diet, its health benefits, and easy recipes that will help you adopt this diet into your lifestyle. The mayr diet is the most common diet used by people who suffer from IBS, as it helps alleviate their symptoms. When you think of the most important organ in your body, what do you think of? Is it your brain, where all your greatest thoughts are created? Perhaps it's your heart, the organ responsible for pumping all the blood that flows through the rest of your body.

What about your stomach? Surely that's up there as one of the things that are important to us. When we're hungry, everything else in the world can seem pretty terrible.

It might seem funny to think that your stomach is one of the most important organs in your body, compared to all the other vital organs, such as the lungs, liver, brain, and heart.

Chapter 1: Breakfast

Classic Western Omelet

Preparation Time: 5 Minutes

Cooking Time: 10 Minutes

Servings: 1

Ingredients:

2 teaspoons coconut oil

3 large eggs, whisked

1 tablespoon heavy cream

Salt and pepper

¼ cup diced green pepper

¼ cup diced yellow onion

¼ cup diced ham

Directions:

In a small bowl, whisk the eggs, heavy cream, salt, and pepper.

Heat up 1 teaspoon of coconut oil over medium heat in a small skillet.

Add the peppers and onions, then sauté the ham for 3 to 4 minutes.

Spoon the mixture in a cup, and heat the skillet with the remaining oil.

Pour in the whisked eggs and cook until the egg's bottom begins to set.

Tilt the pan and cook until almost set to spread the egg.

Spoon the ham and veggie mixture over half of the omelet and turn over.

Let cook the omelet until the eggs are set and then serve hot.

Nutrition:

415 calories,

32,5 g of fat,

25 g of protein,

6,5 g of carbs,

1,5 g of sugar,

5 g of carbs net

Tomato Mozzarella Egg Muffins

Preparation Time: 5 Minutes

Cooking Time: 25 Minutes

Servings: 12

Ingredients:

1 tablespoon butter

1 medium tomato, finely diced

½ cup diced yellow onion

12 large eggs, whisked

½ cup canned coconut milk

¼ cup sliced green onion

Salt and pepper

1 cup shredded mozzarella cheese

Directions:

Preheat the oven to 350 ° F and grease the cooking spray into a muffin pan.

Melt the butter over moderate heat in a medium skillet.

Add the tomato and onions, then cook until softened for 3 to 4 minutes.

Divide the mix between cups of muffins.

Whisk the bacon, coconut milk, green onions, salt, and pepper together and then spoon into the muffin cups.

Sprinkle with cheese until the egg is set, then bake for 15 to 25 minutes.

Nutrition:

135 calories,

10.5 g fat,

9 g protein,

2 g carbs,

0.5 g fiber,

1.5 g net carbs

Crispy Chai Waffles

Preparation Time: 10 Minutes

Cooking Time: 20 Minutes

Servings: 4

Ingredients:

4 large eggs, separated into whites and yolks

3 tablespoons coconut flour

3 tablespoons powdered erythritol

1 ¼ teaspoon baking powder

1 teaspoon vanilla extract

½ teaspoon ground cinnamon

¼ teaspoon ground ginger

Pinch ground cloves

Pinch ground cardamom

3 tablespoons coconut oil, melted

3 tablespoons unsweetened almond milk

Directions:

Divide the eggs into two separate mixing bowls.

Whip the whites of the eggs until stiff peaks develop and then set aside.

Whisk the egg yolks into the other bowl with the coconut flour, erythritol, baking powder, cocoa, cinnamon, cardamom, and cloves.

Pour the melted coconut oil and the almond milk into the second bowl and whisk.

Fold softly in the whites of the egg until you have just combined.

Preheat waffle iron with cooking spray and grease.

Spoon into the iron for about 1/2 cup of batter.

Cook the waffle according to directions from the maker.

Move the waffle to a plate and repeat with the batter left over.

Nutrition:

215 calories,

17 g of fat,

8 g of protein,

8 g of carbohydrates,

4 g of fiber,

4 g of net carbs

Three Cheese Egg Muffins

Preparation Time: 5 Minutes

Cooking Time: 20 Minutes

Servings: 8

Ingredients:

1 tablespoon butter

½ cup diced yellow onion

12 large eggs, whisked

½ cup canned coconut milk

¼ cup sliced green onion

Salt and pepper

½ cup shredded cheddar cheese

½ cup shredded Swiss cheese

¼ cup grated parmesan cheese

Directions:

Preheat the oven to 350 ° F and grease the cooking spray into a muffin pan.

Melt the butter over moderate heat in a medium skillet.

Add the onions then cook until softened for 3 to 4 minutes.

Divide the mix between cups of muffins.

Whisk the bacon, coconut milk, green onions, salt, and pepper together and then spoon into the muffin cups.

In a cup, mix the three kinds of cheese, and scatter over the egg muffins.

Bake till the egg is set, for 20 to 25 minutes.

Nutrition:

150 calories,

11.5 g fat,

10 g protein,

2 g carbs,

0.5 g fiber,

1.5 g net carbs

Anti-Inflammatory Energy Bars

Preparation Time: 15 minutes

Cooking Time: 0 minutes

Servings: 5

Ingredients:

1 ¼ cup packed dates, pitted and chopped

1 cup unsweetened fine coconut meat

1 cup hemp seeds

2/3 cup cashew nuts, toasted and chopped

2 tablespoons coconut oil

Directions:

Place all Ingredients: in a food processor until well-combined.

Line a baking dish with parchment paper and press the dough into the pan.

Place in the fridge for an hour to set.

Once frozen, lift the bars out of the pan and cut into 10 squares.

Nutritional Values:

Calories: 471

Total Fat: 34g

Saturated Fat: 6g

Total Carbs: 41g

Net Carbs: 34g

Protein: 10g

Sugar: 26g

Fiber: 7g

Sodium:60 mg

Potassium 588mg

Leek & Spinach Frittata

Preparation Time: 10 minutes

Cooking Time: 15 minutes

Servings: 4

Ingredients:

2 Leeks, Chopped Fine

2 Tablespoons Avocado Oil

8 Eggs

½ Teaspoon Garlic Powder

½ Teaspoon Bail, Dried

1 Cup Baby Spinach, Fresh & Packed

1 Cup Cremini Mushrooms, Sliced

Sea Salt & Black Pepper to Taste

Directions:

Set the oven to 400°F then get an ovenproof skillet. Place it over medium-high heat, sautéing your leeks in your avocado oil until soft. It should take roughly five minutes

Get out a bowl, and whisk the eggs with your garlic, basil, and salt. Add them to the skillet with your leeks, cooking for five minutes. You'll need to stir frequently.

Stir in your mushrooms and spinach, seasoning with pepper.

Place the skillet in the oven then bake for 10 minutes. Serve warm.

Nutrition:

Calories: 276

Protein: 19 g

Fat: 17 g

Carbs: 15 g

Cherry Chia Oats

Preparation Time: 10 minutes

Cooking Time: 20 minutes

Servings: 2

Ingredients:

¼ Teaspoon Vanilla Extract, Pure

2 Tablespoons Almond Butter

8 Cherries, Fresh, Pitted & Halved

1 Cup Quick Cook Oats

2 Tablespoons Chia Seeds

¼ Cup Whole Milk Yogurt, Plain

1 ¼ Cup Almond Milk

Directions:

Mix all of together the ingredients until they're combined well.

Seal in two jars and refrigerate for twenty-five minutes before serving.

Nutrition:

Calories: 564

Protein: 22 g

Fat: 32 g

Carbs: 27 g

Oven-Poached Eggs

Preparation Time: 2minutes

Cooking Time: 11minutes

Servings: 4

Ingredients:

6 eggs, at room temperature

Water

Ice bath

2 cups water, chilled

2 cups of ice cubes

Directions:

Set the oven to 350°F. Put 2 cups of water into a deep roasting tin, and place it into the lowest rack of the oven.

Place one egg into each cup of cupcake/muffin tins, along with one tablespoon of water.

Carefully place muffin tins into the middle rack of the oven.

Bake eggs for 45 minutes.

Turn off the heat immediately. Take off the muffin tins from the oven and set on a cake rack to cool before extracting eggs.

Pour ice bath ingredients into a large heat-resistant bowl.

Bring the eggs into an ice bath to stop the cooking process. After 10 minutes, drain eggs well. Use as needed.

Nutrition:

Calories: 357 kcal

Protein: 17.14 g

Fat: 24.36 g

Carbohydrates: 16.19 g

Cranberry and Raisins Granola

Preparation Time: 15 minutes

Cooking Time: 20 minutes

Servings: 4

Ingredients:

4 cups old-fashioned rolled oats

1/4 cup sesame seeds

1 cup dried cranberries

1 cup golden raisins

1/8 teaspoon nutmeg

2 tablespoons olive oil

1/2 cup almonds, slivered

2 tablespoons warm water

1 teaspoon vanilla extract

1 teaspoon cinnamon

1/4 teaspoon of salt

6 tablespoons maple syrup

1/3 cup of honey

Directions:

In a bowl, mix the sesame seeds, nutmeg, almonds, oats, salt, and cinnamon.

In another bowl, mix the oil, water, vanilla, honey, and syrup. Gradually pour the mixture into the oats mixture. Toss to combine. Spread the mixture into a greased jelly-roll pan. Bake in the oven at 300°F for at least 55 minutes. Stir and break the clumps every 10 minutes.

Once you get it from the oven, stir the cranberries and raisins. Allow cooling. This will last for a week when stored in an airtight container and up to a month when stored in the fridge.

Nutrition:

Calories: 698 kcal

Protein: 21.34 g

Fat: 20.99 g

Carbohydrates: 148.59 g

Spicy Marble Eggs

Preparation Time: 15 minutes

Cooking Time: 2 hours

Servings: 12

Ingredients:

6 medium-boiled eggs, unpeeled, cooled

For the Marinade

2 oolong black tea bags

3 Tbsp. brown sugar

1 thumb-sized fresh ginger, unpeeled, crushed

3 dried star anise, whole

2 dried bay leaves

3 Tbsp. light soy sauce

4 Tbsp. dark soy sauce

4 cups of water

1 dried cinnamon stick, whole

1 tsp. salt

1 tsp. dried Szechuan peppercorns

Directions:

Using the back of a metal spoon, crack eggshells in places to create a spider web effect. Do not peel. Set aside until needed.

Pour marinade into large Dutch oven set over high heat. Put lid partially on. Bring water to a rolling boil, about 5 minutes. Turn off heat.

Secure lid. Steep ingredients for 10 minutes.

Using a slotted spoon, fish out and discard solids. Cool marinade completely to room proceeding.

Place eggs into an airtight non-reactive container just small enough to snugly fit all these in.

Pour in marinade. Eggs should be completely submerged in liquid. Discard leftover marinade, if any. Line container rim with generous layers of saran wrap. Secure container lid.

Chill eggs for 24 hours before using.

Extract eggs and drain each piece well before using, but keep the rest submerged in the marinade.

Nutrition:

Calories: 75 kcal

Protein: 4.05 g

Fat: 4.36 g

Carbohydrates: 4.83 g

Chapter 2: Lunch

Farro Salad with Arugula

Preparation Time: 10 minutes

Cooking Time: 35 minutes

Servings: 2

Ingredients:

½ cup farro

1 ½ cup chicken stock

1 teaspoon salt

½ teaspoon ground black pepper

2 cups arugula, chopped

1 cucumber, chopped

1 tablespoon lemon juice

½ teaspoon olive oil

½ teaspoon Italian seasoning

Directions:

Mix up together farro, salt, and chicken stock and transfer mixture in the pan.

Close the lid and boil it for 35 minutes.

Meanwhile, place all remaining ingredients in the salad bowl.

Chill the farro to the room temperature and add it in the salad bowl too.

Mix up the salad well.

Nutrition:

Calories 92

Fat 2.3g

Fiber 2g

Carbs 15.6g

Protein 3.9g

Stir-Fried Farros

Preparation Time: 5 minutes

Cooking Time: 35 minutes

Servings: 2

Ingredients:

½ cup farro

1 ½ cup water

1 teaspoon salt

1 teaspoon chili flakes

½ teaspoon paprika

½ teaspoon turmeric

½ teaspoon ground coriander

1 yellow onion, sliced

1 tablespoon butter

1 carrot, grated

Directions:

Place farro in the pan. Add water and salt.

Close the lid and boil it for 30 minutes.

Meanwhile, toss the butter in the skillet.

Heat it and add sliced onion and grated carrot.

Fry the vegetables for 10 minutes over the medium heat. Stir them with the help of spatula from time to time.

When the farro is cooked, add it in the roasted vegetables and mix up well.

Cook stir-fried farro for 5 minutes over the medium-high heat.

Nutritional Values:

Calories 129

Fat 5.9g

Fiber 3g

Carbs 17.1g

Protein 2.8g

Cauliflower Broccoli Mash

Preparation Time: 5 minutes

Cooking Time: 10 minutes

Serving: 6

Ingredients:

1 large head cauliflower, cut into chunks

1 small head broccoli, cut into florets

3 tablespoons extra virgin olive oil

1 teaspoon salt

Pepper, to taste

Directions:

Take a pot and add oil then heat it

Add the cauliflower and broccoli

Season with salt and pepper to taste

Keep stirring to make vegetable soft

Add water if needed

When is already cooked, use a food processor or a potato masher to puree the vegetables

Serve and enjoy!

Nutrition:

Calories: 39

Fat: 3g

Carbohydrates: 2g

Protein: 0.89g

Broccoli and Black Beans Stir Fry

Preparation Time: 10 minutes

Cooking Time: 15 minutes

Servings: 4

Ingredients:

4 cups broccoli florets

1 tablespoon sesame oil

4 teaspoons sesame seeds

2 teaspoons ginger, finely chopped

A pinch turmeric powder

Lime juice to taste (optional)

2 cups cooked black beans

2 cloves garlic, finely minced

A large pinch red chili flakes

Salt to taste

Directions:

Pour enough water to cover the bottom of the saucepan by an inch. Place a strainer on the saucepan. Place broccoli florets on the strainer. Steam the broccoli for 6 minutes.

Place a large frying pan over medium heat. Add sesame oil. When the oil is just warm, add sesame seeds, chili flakes, ginger, garlic, turmeric powder and salt. Sauté for a couple of minutes until aromatic.

Add steamed broccoli and black beans and sauté until thoroughly heated.

Add lime juice and stir.

Serve hot.

Nutrition:

Calories: 196 kcal

Protein: 11.2 g

Fat: 7.25 g

Carbohydrates: 23.45 g

Mushroom "Chicken Tenders"

Prepation Time: 1 hour

Cooking Time: 30 minutes

Servings: 6

Ingredients:

- Grapeseed oil as needed
- 1 tsp. ground cloves
- 1 tsp. cayenne powder
- 2 tsp. ginger powder
- 2 tsp. onion powder
- 2 tsp. sage
- 2 tsp sea salt

2 tsp. basil

2 tsp. oregano

1 ½ cup spelt flour

1 ½ cups spring flour

2 to 6 Portobello mushrooms

Directions:

Slice the mushrooms caps approximately half-inch apart.

Add mushrooms, oil, water, and half of the individual seasonings to the bowl and mix for 1 hour.

In a separate bowl, blend the rest of the seasonings and the spelt flour and then batter the mushrooms.

Preheat oven to 400F. Grease a baking sheet with grapeseed oil and put the mushrooms on the baking sheet. Bake 15 minutes per side, or until crispy. Serve.

Nutritional Values:

Calories: 276

Fat: 6.5g

Carb: 49.48g

Protein: 10.72g

Quinoa Pasta with Tomato Artichoke Sauce

Prepation Time: 10 minutes

Cooking Time: 20 minutes

Servings: 2

Ingredients:

    2 tbsp extra-virgin olive oil

    1 pinch cayenne pepper

    ½ tsp. sea salt

    3 tbsp. basil, fresh

    1 tsp. vegetable stock

    1-ounce walnuts

    1 fennel bulb

    1 onion, chopped

    8 ounces artichoke hearts

    5 ounces cherry tomatoes, fresh

7 ounces quinoa or spelt pasta

Directions:

Cook the artichoke until tender. Then cook the pasta as stated in the package directions. Chopped all the veggies.

Heat 2 tablespoons of oil then stir fry onions, nuts, and fennel for a few minutes. Then add the cooked artichokes and tomatoes and cook for 2 minutes.

Scoop about ½ cup of water and then dissolve the vegetable stock into the water. Add into a pan and simmer for 2 minutes on low heat. Stir regularly.

Add basil, season with salt and pepper. Put the sauce on the pasta and serve.

Nutritional Values:

Calories: 719

Fat: 26g

Carb: 111g

Protein: 23.9g

Alkalizing Tahini Noodle Bowl

Prepation Time: 10 minutes

Cooking Time: 0 minutes

Servings: 2

Ingredients:

   1 tsp. black sesame seeds

   ½ avocado, chopped

   2 green onions, chopped

   4 kale, chopped

   1 parsnip, shredded

   4 leaves of romaine, chopped

   1 yellow zucchini, spiralized

Dressing:

   1 tsp. agave

   2 tbsp. lemon juice

   1 tbsp. tahini

Dash of salt

Directions:

Put all the vegetables you chopped in a bowl. Add all ingredients for dressing in another bowl and whisk.

Put the dressing over the vegetables then garnish with sesame seeds.

Nutritional Values:

Calories: 209

Fat: 14.5g

Carb: 22.07g

Protein: 5.49g

Roasted Vegetables

Preparation Time: 14 minutes

Cooking Time: 17 minutes

Servings: 3

Ingredients:

4 Tbsp. olive oil, reserve some for greasing

2 heads, large garlic, tops sliced off

2 large eggplants/aubergine, tops removed, cubed

2 large shallots, peeled, quartered

1 large carrot, peeled, cubed

1 large parsnips, peeled, cubed

1 small green bell pepper, deseeded, ribbed, cubed

1 small red bell pepper, deseeded, ribbed, cubed

½ pound Brussels sprouts, halved, do not remove cores

1 sprig, large thyme, leaves picked

sea salt, coarse-grained

For garnish:

1 large lemon, halved, ½ squeezed, ½ sliced into smaller wedges

1/8 cup fennel bulb, minced

Directions:

Heat up oven to 425°F or 220°C for at least 5 minutes before using.

Line deep roasting pan with aluminum foil; lightly grease with oil. Tumble in bell peppers, Brussels sprouts, carrots, eggplants, garlic, parsnips, rosemary leaves, shallots, and thyme. Add a pinch of sea salt; drizzle in remaining oil and lemon juice. Toss well to combine.

Cover roasting pan with a sheet of aluminum foil. Place this on middle rack of oven. Bake for 20 to 30 minutes. Remove aluminum foil. Roast for extra 5 to 10 minutes, or until some vegetables brown at the edges. Remove roasting pan from oven. Cool slightly before ladling equal portions into plates.

Garnish with fennel and a wedge of lemon. Squeeze lemon juice on top of dish before eating.

Nutritional Values:

Calories 163

Total Fat 4.2 g

Saturated Fat 0.8 g

Cholesterol 0 mg

Sodium 861 mg

Total Carbs 22.5 g

Fiber 6.3 g

Sugar 2.3 g

Protein 9.2 g

Sweet and Sour Onions

Preparation Time: 10 minutes

Cooking Time: 11 minutes

Servings: 4

Ingredients:

 4 large onions, halved

 2 garlic cloves, crushed

 3 cups vegetable stock

 1 ½ tablespoon balsamic vinegar

 ½ teaspoon Dijon mustard

 1 tablespoon sugar

Directions:

Combine onions and garlic in a pan. Fry for 3 minutes, or till softened.

Pour stock, vinegar, Dijon mustard, and sugar. Bring to a boil.

Reduce heat. Cover and let the mix simmer for 10 minutes.

Remove from heat. Continue stirring until the liquid is reduced and the onions are brown. Serve.

Nutritional Values:

Calories 203

Total Fat 41.2 g

Saturated Fat 0.8 g

Cholesterol 0 mg

Sodium 861 mg

Total Carbs 29.5 g

Fiber 16.3 g

Sugar 29.3 g

Protein 19.2 g

Sautéed Apples and Onions

Preparation Time: 14 minutes

Cooking Time: 16 minutes

Servings: 3

Ingredients:

    2 cups dry cider

    1 large onion, halved

    2 cups vegetable stock

    4 apples, sliced into wedges

    Pinch of salt

    Pinch of pepper

Directions:

Combine cider and onion in a saucepan. Bring to a boil until the onions are cooked and liquid almost gone.

Pour the stock and the apples. Season with salt and pepper. Stir occasionally. Cook for 10 minutes or you may wait until the apples are tender but not mushy. Serve.

Nutritional Values:

Calories 343

Total Fat 51.2 g

Saturated Fat 0.8 g

Cholesterol 0 mg

Sodium 861 mg

Total Carbs 22.5 g

Fiber 6.3 g

Sugar 2.3 g

Protein 9.2 g

Zucchini Noodles with Portabella Mushrooms

Preparation Time: 14 minutes

Cooking Time: 16 minutes

Servings: 3

Ingredients:

- 1 zucchini, processed into spaghetti-like noodles
- 3 garlic cloves, minced
- 2 white onions, thinly sliced
- 1 thumb-sized ginger, julienned

1 lb. chicken thighs

1 lb. portabella mushrooms, sliced into thick slivers

2 cups chicken stock

3 cups water

Pinch of sea salt, add more if needed

Pinch of black pepper, add more if needed

2 tsp. sesame oil

4 Tbsp. coconut oil, divided

¼ cup fresh chives, minced, for garnish

Directions:

Begin by pouring 2 tablespoons of coconut oil into a large saucepan. Fry mushroom slivers in batches for 5 minutes or until seared brown. Set aside. Transfer these to a plate.

Sauté onion, ginger, and garlic for 3 minutes or until tender. Add in chicken thighs, cooked mushrooms, chicken stock, water, salt, and pepper stir mixture well. Bring to a boil.

Lessen heat then allow to simmer for 20 minutes or until the chicken is fork tender. Tip in sesame oil.

Serve by placing an equal amount of zucchini noodles into bowls. Ladle soup and garnish with chives.

Nutritional Values:

Calories 163

Total Fat 4.2 g

Saturated Fat 0.8 g

Cholesterol 0 mg

Sodium 861 mg

Total Carbs 22.5 g

Fiber 6.3 g

Sugar 2.3 g

Protein 9.2 g

Grilled Tempeh with Pineapple

Preparation Time: 12 minutes

Cooking Time: 16 minutes

Servings: 3

Ingredients:

10 oz. tempeh, sliced

1 red bell pepper, quartered

1/4 pineapple, sliced into rings

6 oz. green beans

1 tbsp. coconut aminos

2 1/2 tbsp. orange juice, freshly squeeze

1 1/2 tbsp. lemon juice, freshly squeezed

1 tbsp. extra virgin olive oil

1/4 cup hoisin sauce

Directions:

Mix the olive oil, lemon, and orange juices, coconut aminos or soy sauce, and hoisin sauce in a bowl. Add the diced tempeh and set aside.

Heat up the grill or place a grill pan over medium high flame. Once hot, lift the marinated tempeh from the bowl with a pair of tongs and transfer them to the grill or pan.

Grill for 2 to 3 minutes, or wait until browned all over.

Grill the sliced pineapples alongside the tempeh, then transfer them directly onto the serving platter.

Place the grilled tempeh beside the grilled pineapple and cover with aluminum foil to keep warm.

Meanwhile, place the green beans and bell peppers in a bowl and add just enough of the marinade to coat.

Prepare the grill pan and add the vegetables. Grill until fork tender and slightly charred.

Transfer the grilled vegetables to the serving platter and arrange artfully with the tempeh and pineapple. Serve at once.

Nutritional Values:

Calories 163

Total Fat 4.2 g

Saturated Fat 0.8 g

Cholesterol 0 mg

Sodium 861 mg

Total Carbs 22.5 g

Fiber 6.3 g

Sugar 2.3 g

Protein 9.2 g

Alkaline Meatloaf

Preparation time: 15 minutes

Cooking time: 70 minutes

Servings: 1 loaf

Ingredients:

    1 cup prepared wild rice

    ½ cup homemade tomato sauce, divided

    ½ cup chopped yellow onion, divided

    ½ cup chopped green bell pepper, divided

    1 shallot, chopped

    2 cups mixed mushrooms, chopped

    ¼ tsp. cloves

    ½ tsp. ginger

    ½ tsp. tarragon

    1 tsp. thyme

1 tsp. sage

1 tbsp. sea salt

1 tbsp. onion powder

1 cup garbanzo flour or spelt flour

cups breadcrumbs (made of spelt flour)

2 cups cooked chickpeas

Cayenne to taste

Directions:

Clean and dry wild rice. Prepare the chickpeas as well and set them aside.

Mix garbanzo flour or spelt flour with bread crumbs and set the mixture aside.

Chop the green peppers and the onions and place half of each of them to the side.

Now chop the shallots and mushrooms and add them to a food processor, along with chickpeas, half of the onion, half of the green peppers, and spices.

Pulse the mixture until fully incorporated. Then add in 2 tbsp of tomato sauce and the wild rice. And continue to blend until a paste.

Move the mixture to a mixing bowl. Add the remaining flour, bread crumbs, onion, and green pepper. Mix well.

Pour the mixture into a greased pan and cover with the remaining tomato sauce—Bake in the preheated oven at 350F within 60 to 70 minutes. Cool, slice, and serve.

Nutritional Values:

Calories: 265

Fat: 2.96g

Carb: 48g

Protein: 13.15g

Chapter 3: Dinner Recipes

Italian Leek Fry

Preparation Time: 10minutes

Cooking Time: 20 minutes

Serving: 2

Ingredients:

2 silvered stalks of leeks

2 diced up middle sized white onion

1 silvered Zucchini

2 coarsely diced up tomatoes

2 tablespoon of extra virgin olive oil

1 tablespoon of grated cheddar

1 teaspoon of sea salt

1 tablespoon of parsley

1 teaspoon of oregano

½ a teaspoon of curry powder

Freshly ground black pepper

½ a cup of water

Directions:

Take a medium sized pan and add olive oil, heat it up over medium heat. Add onions and sauté them until lightly browned. Add zucchinis and cook for about 3-4 minutes

Pour water and cover up the pan. Lower down the heat to low and let it simmer for 10 minutes

Add tomatoes and season with some pepper and curry powder. Cook for 10 minutes, making sure to keep the lid closed. Once done, season with some more parsley and salt. Add cheese and serve! Serve with some bread if you require your meal to have greater alkaline value!

Nutrition:

80 Calories

7g Fats

4g Carbs

1g Fiber

Bell Peppers & Zucchini Stir Fry

Preparation Time: 15 minutes

Cooking Time: 15 minutes

Servings: 4

Ingredients:

2 tablespoons avocado oil

1 large onion, cubed

4 garlic cloves, minced

1 large green bell pepper

1 large red bell pepper

1 large yellow bell pepper

2 cups zucchini, sliced

¼ cup spring water

Sea salt, as required

Cayenne powder, as required

Directions:

Cook the oil over medium heat and sauté the onion and garlic for about 4-5 minutes. Add the vegetables and stir fry for about 4-5 minutes. Add the water and stir fry for about 3-4 minutes more. Serve hot.

Nutritional Values:

66 Calories

1.3g Total Fat

2.3g Protein

13.5g Carbs

3g Fiber

Yellow Squash & Bell Pepper Bake

Preparation Time: 15 minutes

Cooking Time: 20 minutes

Servings: 4

Ingredients:

2 large yellow squash

1 large red bell pepper

1 large yellow bell peppers

1 onion, cubed

1 tablespoon agave nectar

2 tablespoons grapeseed oil

1 teaspoon cayenne powder

Sea salt, as required

Directions:

Lightly, grease the baking dish and preheat the oven to 375 degrees. Mix all the ingredients in a bowl. Transfer the vegetable mixture into the prepared baking dish. Bake for about 15-20 minutes. Remove from the oven and serve immediately.

Nutritional Values:

132 Calories

7.6g Total Fat

2.9g Protein

16.7g Carbs

3.5g Fiber

Vegetable Medley Sauté

Preparation Time: 10 minutes

Cooking Time: 15 minutes

Serving: 4

Ingredients:

1 cup mushrooms (sliced)

1 zucchini (sliced)

1 yellow squash (sliced)

1 red pepper (chopped)

1 green pepper (chopped)

2 plum tomatoes (chopped)

½ red onion (finely chopped)

½ cup chayote (finely chopped)

3 tbsp. grape-seed oil or avocado oil

⅛ tsp cayenne pepper

⅛ tsp sea salt

Directions:

Cook the oil in a saucepan over medium heat. Let the oil get hot. Add in mushrooms and onions and sauté for 4 minutes. Add in the rest of the vegetables and spices and sauté for 8-10 minutes.

Nutrition:

115 calories

4.9g fiber

21g protein

Chickpea Butternut Squash

Preparation Time: 10 minutes

Cooking Time: 15 minutes

Serving: 2

Ingredients:

15 oz. cooked chickpeas

1 ½ section of a butternut squash

¼ plum tomato

¼ cup coconut milk

1 cup water (add more water to make thinner soup)

Pinch of dill

Pinch of all spice

Pinch of cayenne pepper

⅛ tsp of sea salt

Directions:

Add all the ingredients to a blender and blend to your desired consistency. Add the blended ingredients to a saucepan over a medium/high flame until it starts to boil or air bubbles rise. Adjust it into low heat and cook for 30 minutes.

Nutrition:

110 calories

9.7g fiber

11g protein

Grilled Vegetable Stack

Preparation Time: 10 minutes

Cooking Time: 20 minutes

Servings: 2

Ingredients:

    1/2 zucchini, sliced into slices about 1/4-inch thick

    2 stemmed Portobello mushrooms with the gills removed

    1 tsp. divided sea salt

    1/2 cup divided hummus

    1 peeled and sliced red onion

    1 seeded red bell pepper, sliced lengthwise

    1 seeded yellow bell pepper, sliced lengthwise

Directions:

    Adjust the temperature of your broiler or grill.

    Grill the mushroom caps over coal or gas flame.

    Add the yellow and red bell peppers, onion, and zucchini for about 20 minutes as you turn it occasionally.

Fill the mushroom cap with 1/4 cup of hummus.

Top it with some onion, yellow peppers, red and zucchini.

Add salt to season then set it aside.

Repeat the process with the second mushroom cap and the remaining ingredients.

Serve.

Nutritional Values:

Calories: 179

Fat: 3.1g

Carbs: 15.7g

Protein: 3.9g

Date Night Chive Bake

Preparation Time: 10 minutes

Cooking Time: 30 minutes

Servings: 2

Ingredients:

    4 peeled and sliced lengthwise zucchinis

1 lb. Radish chopped into bite-size pieces

2 tsps. Seville orange zest

3 peeled and chopped chive heads cloves

2 tbsps. Coconut oil

1 cup vegetable broth

1/4 tsps. Mustard powder

1 tsp. sea salt

Directions:

Adjust the temperature of the oven to 400°F.

In a separate bowl, mix all the ingredients.

Spread the mixture in a baking pan evenly.

Cover the mixture with a piece of aluminum foil then place it in the oven.

Bake the mixture for about 30 minutes as you stir it once halfway through the cook time.

Serve.

Nutritional Values:

Calories: 270

Fat: 15.2g

Carbs: 28.1g

Protein: 11.6g

Curried Zucchini

Preparation Time: 5 minutes

Cooking Time: 5 minutes

Servings: 2

Ingredients:

    Cooked quinoa

    Flesh roasted zucchini

    Water

    1 tsp. curry powder

    1 tsp. sea salt

    1 tsp. sesame oil

    1 Seville orange juice

Directions:

In the food processor, mix the salt, zucchini, sesame oil, seville orange juice, and curry powder.

Blend the mixture until it becomes smooth.

In a saucepan over moderate heat, transfer zucchini mixture then warm it for 5 minutes.

Add a little water to thin it.

Serve over the cooked quinoa.

Serve.

Nutritional Values:

Calories: 81

Fat: 81g

Carbs: 14.1g

Protein: 2.4g

Chapter 4: Salads

Buckwheat Salad

Preparation Time: 10 minutes

Cooking Time: 15 minutes

Servings: 2

Ingredients:

1 cup raw buckwheat, rinsed

2 cups water

2 handfuls fresh baby spinach leaves, rinsed

Handful fresh basil leaves, rinsed

2 scallions, white parts only, rinsed and chopped

Zest of 1 lemon

Juice of ½ lemon

½ red onion, finely chopped

Himalayan pink salt

Freshly ground black pepper

¼ cup extra-virgin olive oil

1 red chili, rinsed and thinly sliced

2 tablespoons mixed sprouts, rinsed

1 ripe avocado, peeled, pitted, and sliced

1½ ounces feta cheese (optional)

Direction:

Mix the buckwheat and water, then bring it to boil over high heat. Reduce the heat to simmer and cook for 15 minutes, or until soft. Remove from the heat and let cool.

Meanwhile, in a food processor, combine the baby spinach, basil, scallions, lemon zest, and lemon juice, and process for 30 seconds. Stir the herb mixture into the cooled buckwheat.

Add the red onion and season with salt and pepper. Arrange the buckwheat on a platter. Drizzle with the olive oil and scatter on the chopped chili and sprouts. Top with the sliced avocado, crumble the feta over top (if using), and serve.

Nutrition:

685 calories

54g total fat

43g total carbohydrates

16g fiber

5g sugar

Mixed Sprouts Salad

Preparation Time: 10 minutes

Cooking Time: 0 minute

Servings: 2

Ingredients:

1 to 2 tablespoons coconut oil

Juice of 1 lemon

Handful fresh chives, rinsed and chopped

Handful fresh dill, rinsed and chopped

Handful fresh parsley, rinsed and chopped

½ teaspoon Himalayan pink salt

½ teaspoon freshly ground black pepper

1 scallion, rinsed and chopped

1 cucumber, rinsed and chopped

½ cup mixed sprouts of choice (alfalfa, radish, broccoli, mung bean, cress, etc.), rinsed

Directions:

In a blender, combine the coconut oil, lemon juice, chives, dill, parsley, salt, and pepper, and blend until mainly smooth. Transfer to a medium bowl. Stir in the scallion, cucumber, and sprouts to coat, and serve.

Nutrition:

168 calories

14g total fat

12g total carbohydrates

1g fiber

4g sugar

Thai Quinoa Salad

Preparation Time: 15 minutes

Cooking Time: 0 minute

Servings: 2

Ingredients:

For the Dressing

⅓ cup filtered water

¼ cup tahini

1 pitted date

1 tablespoon sesame seeds

1 tablespoon apple cider vinegar

2 teaspoons tamari

1 teaspoon freshly squeezed lemon juice

1 teaspoon toasted sesame oil

1 teaspoon chopped garlic

½ teaspoon Himalayan pink salt

For the Salad

1 cup quinoa, rinsed and steamed

1 cup arugula, rinsed and chopped

1 tomato, rinsed and sliced

¼ red onion, rinsed and diced

Directions:

To Make the Dressing

Blend the water, tahini, date, sesame seeds, vinegar, tamari, lemon juice, sesame oil, garlic, and salt on high speed until smooth.

To Make the Salad

Combine together the quinoa, arugula, tomato, and red onion. Drizzle the dressing, toss it well to coat, and serve.

Nutrition:

558 calories

25g total fat

69g total carbohydrates

10g fiber

4g sugar

19g protein

Sweet Potato Salad

Preparation Time: 15 minutes

Cooking Time: 5 minutes

serves 2

Ingredients:

For the Dressing

½ cup sesame oil

2 tablespoons coconut oil

2 tablespoons light soy sauce

1 tablespoon coconut sugar or raw honey

1 garlic clove, crushed

For the Salad

5½ ounces fresh baby spinach leaves, rinsed

1 red onion, rinsed and finely chopped

1 tomato, rinsed, seeded, and chopped

1 tablespoon coconut oil

1 large sweet potato, scrubbed, peeled, and diced

Directions:

To Make the Dressing

In a small bowl, whisk the sesame oil, coconut oil, soy sauce, coconut sugar, and garlic until blended. Set aside.

To Make the Salad

In a large salad bowl, gently toss together the baby spinach, red onion, and tomato. Set aside.

In a small skillet over medium heat, heat the coconut oil. Add the sweet potato and cook for 3 to 5 minutes, stirring, until golden brown. Using a slotted spoon, add the sweet potato to the salad and gently stir to combine. Pour the dressing over the salad, gently toss again to coat, and serve.

Nutrition:

550 calories

52g total fat

20g total carbohydrates

3g fiber

9g sugar

Waldorf Salad

Preparation Time: 15 minutes plus overnight to soak

Cooking Time: 0 minute

Servings: 2

Ingredients:

For the Dressing

1 ripe avocado, peeled and pitted

1 teaspoon Dijon mustard

½ teaspoon Himalayan pink salt

Freshly ground black pepper

Juice of ½ lemon

For the Salad

2 cups canned chickpeas, rinsed and drained, or cooked, drained, and cooled

1 cup sunflower seeds, soaked in filtered water overnight, drained

2 apples, rinsed, cored, and chopped

½ red onion, rinsed and diced

1 celery stalk, rinsed and diced

1 to 2 teaspoons chopped fresh dill, rinsed

Directions:

To Make the Dressing

In a small bowl, using a fork, mash together the avocado, mustard, salt, pepper, and lemon juice. Set aside.

To Make the Salad

In a large bowl, stir together the chickpeas, sunflower seeds, and dressing until well combined. Stir in the apples, red onion, and celery. Top with the fresh dill and serve.

Nutrition:

700 calories

40g total fat

80g total carbohydrates

28g fiber

28g protein

Italian Roasted Vegetable Salad

Preparation Time: 15 minutes

Cooking Time: 25 minutes

Servings: 2

Ingredients:

1 cup mushrooms, rinsed and chopped

1 zucchini, rinsed and chopped

1 red onion, rinsed and sliced

1 yellow squash, rinsed and cut into medium chunks

1 green bell pepper, rinsed and cut into thin strips

1 red bell pepper, rinsed and cut into thin strips

3 tablespoons extra-virgin olive oil

1½ teaspoons Italian seasoning

½ teaspoon Himalayan pink salt

¼ teaspoon freshly ground black pepper

1 teaspoon dried parsley

Directions:

Preheat the oven to 425°F. Line a large baking sheet with parchment paper and set aside.

In a large bowl, combine the mushrooms, zucchini, red onion, yellow squash, and green and red bell peppers. Drizzle the olive oil over the veggies and stir to mix well.

Add the Italian seasoning, salt, pepper, and parsley, and stir well again until fully mixed. Spread the veggies on the prepared baking sheet in a single layer.

Roast for 25 minutes, stirring the vegetables halfway through the cooking time, or until tender.

Nutrition:

270 calories

20g total fat

18g total carbohydrates

6g fiber

10g sugar

5g protein

Kale and Carrot Salad

Preparation Time: 15 minutes

Cooking Time: 0 minutes

Serving: 5

Ingredients:

0.6 lb. kale leaves, chopped

2 tbsp. lime juice

4 tbsp. olive oil

salt and ground black pepper to taste

2 carrots, peeled, shredded

0.3 lb. red cabbage, shredded

1 small red onion, chopped

1 garlic clove, minced

Directions:

Combine kale leaves, carrots, cabbage, onion, and garlic. Mix in salt, pepper, lime juice, and olive oil. Toss to combine. Add to a serving bowl.

Nutritional Values:

241 Calories

5g Fat

42g Carbohydrates

4g Protein

Cauliflower and Cherry Tomato Salad

Preparation Time: 15 minutes

Cooking Time: 0 minutes

Servings: 4

Ingredients:

1 head cauliflower

2 tablespoons parsley

2 cups cherry tomatoes, halved

2 tablespoons lemon juice, fresh

2 tablespoons pine nuts

Directions:

Blend lemon juice, cherry tomatoes, cauliflower and parsley then season. Garnish with pine nuts, and mix well before serving.

Nutritional Values:

Calories 64

Protein 2.8g

Fat 3.3g

Watermelon Salad

Preparation Time: 18 minutes

Cooking Time: 0 minute

Servings: 6

Ingredients:

¼ teaspoon sea salt

¼ teaspoon black pepper

1 tablespoon balsamic vinegar

1 cantaloupe, quartered & seeded

12 watermelon, small & seedless

2 cups mozzarella balls, fresh

1/3 cup basil, fresh & torn

2 tablespoons olive oil

Directions:

Scoop out balls of cantaloupe, and the put them in a colander over bowl.

With a melon baller slice the watermelon.

Allow your fruit to drain for ten minutes, and then refrigerate the juice.

Wipe the bowl dry, and then place your fruit in it.

Stir in basil, oil, vinegar, mozzarella and tomatoes before seasoning.

Mix well and serve.

Nutrition:

Calories 218

Protein 10g

Fat 13g

Orange Celery Salad

Preparation Time: 16 minutes

Cooking Time: 0 minute

Servings: 6

Size/ Portion: 2 cups

Ingredients:

1 tablespoon lemon juice, fresh

¼ teaspoon sea salt, fine

¼ teaspoon black pepper

1 tablespoon olive brine

1 tablespoon olive oil

¼ cup red onion, sliced

½ cup green olives

2 oranges, peeled & sliced

3 celery stalks, sliced diagonally in ½ inch slices

Directions:

Put your oranges, olives, onion and celery in a shallow bowl.

Stir oil, olive brine and lemon juice, pour this over your salad.

Season with salt and pepper before serving.

Nutrition:

Calories 65

Protein 2g

Fat 0.2g

Cauliflower & Tomato Salad

Preparation Time: 17 minutes

Cooking Time: 0 minute

Servings: 4

Ingredients:

1 Head Cauliflower, Chopped

2 Tablespoons Parsley, Fresh & chopped

2 Cups Cherry Tomatoes, Halved

2 Tablespoons Lemon Juice, Fresh

2 Tablespoons Pine Nuts

Directions:

Incorporate lemon juice, cherry tomatoes, cauliflower and parsley and season well. Sprinkle the pine nuts, and mix.

Nutrition:

Calories 64

Protein 2.8g

Fat 3.3g

Chapter 5: Desserts and Snacks

Watermelon Sorbet

Preparation Time: 5 minutes

Cooking Time: 15 minutes

Servings: 4

Ingredients:

1 Seedless Watermelon, cubed

Directions:

To start with, place the watermelon cubes in a baking sheet in an even layer.

After that, keep the sheet in the freezer for 2 hours or until the watermelon is solid.

Next, transfer the frozen watermelon cubes in the high-speed blender and puree them until you get a smooth puree.

Then, pour the puree among the two loaf pans.

 Nutrition:

Calories: 427Kcal

Proteins:5.9g

Carbohydrates: 80g

Fat: 15.6g

Almond Butter Balls Vegan

Preparation Time: 10 minutes

Cooking Time: 0 0 minute

Servings: 4

Ingredients:

12 dates, pitted and diced

1/3 cup of unsweetened shredded coconut

2 and a ½ tablespoon of almond butter

Directions:

Take a bowl and add dates, almond butter, and coconut

Mix well

Use the mixture to form small balls

Store them in your fridge and chill them

Enjoy!

Nutrition:

Calories: 62 Cal

Fats: 3 g

Carbohydrates:8 g

Protein:1 g

Coffee Cream

Preparation Time: 10 minutes

Cooking Time: 15 minutes

Servings: 4

Ingredients:

¼ cup brewed coffee

2 tablespoons swerve

2 cups heavy cream

1 teaspoon vanilla extract

2 tablespoons ghee, melted

2 eggs

Directions:

In a bowl, combine the coffee with the cream and the other ingredients, whisk well and divide it into 4 ramekins and whisk well.

Introduce the ramekins in the oven at 350 degrees F and bake for 15 minutes.

Serve warm.

Nutrition:

Calories 300

Fat: 11g

Carbohydrates: 3g

 Protein: 4g

Sugar: 12g

Almond Cookies

Preparation Time: 15 minutes

Cooking Time: 15 minutes

Servings: 12

Ingredients:

14oz / 400g non-wheat flour

1tsp baking soda

1tsp baking powder

3.5oz / 100g tahini

1.7oz / 50g coconut butter

½ tsp vanilla

½ tsp honey

Salt

Directions:

Mix the flour, soda, salt, baking powder together.

Mix tahini and coconut butter together and add 2 tbsp water in the same bowl.

Add honey, vanilla to the tahini mixture and blend it well with a mixer.

Preheat your oven (180C/356F) and put a baking sheet on it.

Add 24 tablespoons of the mixture onto the baking sheet and let it bake in the oven for 11-15 minutes.

Let it get cold a little bit and serve.

Nutrition:

Calories: 112

Carbohydrates:18 g

Protein: 3.2 g

Fat: 1.6 g

Sugar: 23.1 g

Fiber: 7.4 g

Sodium: 28 mg

Chocolate Mousse

Preparation Time: 10 minutes

Cooking Time: 0 minute

Servings: 4

Ingredients:

Coconut cream scraped from the upper side of 2 pieces of 13.5-ounce chilled cans of full-fat coconut milk

4 tablespoons of cocoa

3 tablespoons of Agave Nectar

1 teaspoon of vanilla extract

Directions:

Take a large bowl and scoop out the thick coconut cream from the can to the bowl

Add nectar, vanilla extract and cocoa to the bowl

Beat it well using an electric mixer, starting from low and going to medium until a foamy texture appears

Divide the mix evenly amongst ramekins and chill to your desired level of cold

Enjoy!

Nutrition:

Calories: 134 Cal

Fat: 3.8 g

Carbohydrates: 16 g

Protein: 3.8 g

Strawberry Granita

Preparation Time: 10 minutes

Cooking Time: 10 minutes

Servings: 8

Ingredients:

2 lb. strawberries, halved & hulled

1 cup of water

Agave to taste

¼ teaspoon balsamic vinegar

½ teaspoon lemon juice

Just a small pinch of salt

Directions:

Rinse the strawberries in water.

Keep in a blender. Add water, agave, balsamic vinegar, salt, and lemon juice.

Pulse many times so that the mixture moves. Blend to make it smooth.

Pour into a baking dish. The puree should be 3/8 inch deep only.

Refrigerate the dish uncovered till the edges start to freeze. The center should be slushy.

Stir crystals from the edges lightly into the center. Mix thoroughly.

Chill till the granite is almost completely frozen.

Scrape loose the crystals like before and mix.

Refrigerate again. Use a fork to stir 3-4 times till the granite has become light.

Nutrition:

Calories 72

Carbohydrates 17g

Fat 0g

Sugar 14g

Fiber 2g

Protein 1g

Apple Fritters

Preparation Time: 15 minutes

Cooking Time: 10 minutes

Servings: 4

Ingredients:

1 apple, cored, peeled, and chopped

1 cup all-purpose flour

1 egg

½ cup cashew milk

1-1/2 teaspoons of baking powder

2 tablespoons of stevia sugar

Directions:

Preheat your air fryer to 175 degrees C or 350 degrees F.

Keep parchment paper at the bottom of your fryer.

Apply cooking spray.

Mix together ¼ cup sugar, flour, baking powder, egg, milk, and salt in a bowl.

Combine well by stirring.

Sprinkle 2 tablespoons of sugar on the apples. Coat well.

Combine the apples into your flour mixture.

Use a cookie scoop and drop the fritters with it to the air fryer basket's bottom.

Now air fry for 5 minutes.

Flip the fritters once and fry for another 3 minutes. They should be golden.

Nutritional Values:

Calories 307

Carbohydrates 65g

Cholesterol 48mg

Total Fat 3g

Protein 5g

Sugar 39g

Fiber 2g

Sodium 248mg

Chocolate Mousse

Preparation Time: 10 minutes

Cooking Time: 0 minutes

Servings: 4

Ingredients:

Coconut cream scraped from the upper side of 2 pieces of 13.5-ounce chilled cans of full-fat coconut milk

4 tablespoons of cocoa

3 tablespoons of Agave Nectar

1 teaspoon of vanilla extract

Directions:

Take a large bowl and scoop out the thick coconut cream from the can to the bowl

Add nectar, vanilla extract and cocoa to the bowl

Beat it well using an electric mixer, starting from low and going to medium until a foamy texture appears

Divide the mix evenly amongst ramekins and chill to your desired level of cold

Enjoy!

Nutrition:

Calories: 134 Cal

Fat: 3.8 g

Carbohydrates: 16 g

Protein: 3.8 g

Conclusion

My wish is that you are able to experience a much more comfortable life with the information and recipes from this book and that you are able to eat to your heart's content without worrying about painful or embarrassing symptoms. I hope you are able to find a safe ground with these recipes and that you get to experience a whole new world of IBS treatment. It is hard to believe it's taken people so long to make the connection between good gut health and their overall wellbeing. After all, no other system is so integrally involved in fueling your body, or so literally intertwined with everything inside your body. Poor gut health and an imbalance in the gut microbiome have been linked to everything from arthritis to cancer and heart disease, to poor immune function. It can make you absent-minded or moody, and it can cause you to gain weight and have trouble losing it. It may even be causing or worsening imperfections in your skin.You are also aware of the damage poor diet and some of the choices you make can cause to your gut and entire system. You now realize the importance of the gut not only to your physical health, but to your mental health and mood as well. However, this is just the tip of the iceberg. If eating certain foods can keep everyone healthy then there will be no disease or disorders in the world. The body is a system and when there is an ailment, the entire system suffers, so it is a good idea to find the root and address it. It is also important to treat the body as the system that it is during the healing process.Besides proper diet and balancing gut flora, there are other things you can do to maintain good digestive health. All types of new dietary plans take some getting used to and a little bit of willpower, but remember, this plan is not meant to restrict your calories or the pleasure you gain from sharing food with friends or family. It is meant instead to help you enjoy food without painful side effects. Keep this in mind during those times when temptation starts to pop in. The recipes included in this book have been designed to be simple and delicious. My hope is that this will help you keep on track with your dietary goals.

Finally, embrace the change that you are making with your body. You are taking charge of your health and regaining control of your life, both of which are truly wonderful things.

CPSIA information can be obtained
at www.ICGtesting.com
Printed in the USA
LVHW051552300621
691578LV00003B/89